Digestive Herbs

With Recipes according to Hildegard von Bingen

Table of Contents

"No tree greens without strength to green,

no stone lacks green moisture,

no creature is without these qualities;

living eternity itself is not

without this power to green."

- Hildegard von Bingen -

Foreword

Studying herbalism is a journey through the history of mankind. Since their evolutionary beginnings as hunter-gatherers, humans have made considerable progress in botany and the use of health-promoting plant extracts.

It is striking that plant-based food has usually been more than just a food basis throughout the ages. There was no strict separation between food and medicine, as is customary for today's pharmacology. Rather, health problems were prevented by the daily diet.

In this context, herbalists, botanists and physicians together set the tone and bequeathed to the peoples of the world a wealth of knowledge for maintaining health thanks to their detailed records of the ingredients, effects and preparation of plant-based foods.

One name that is difficult to avoid in the field of healthy nutrition is Hildegard von Bingen. A spiritual cult figure of the Middle Ages, who has even been awarded as a saint since 2012. However, Hildegard's religious status as a Benedictine nun and abbess hardly does her work justice.

It may seem a bit controversial at first glance, but one of the most important clergymen of the Roman Catholic Church is also a dignitary of the pagan tradition and in particular a style icon of modern herb women.

In many a witch's shelf, among writings on pagan customs and witchcraft, there is also one or the other book about the healing art of Hildegard von Bingen. If the rumours are to be believed, Hildegard herself was even a "witch woman" who only survived at the time of the witch hunts because she quietly pursued her herbal witchcraft behind German monastery walls. This would not be difficult to imagine with a woman who was considered the most important mystic, poet and feminist of antiquity.

In many respects, Hildegard broke completely new ground, which did not always conform to the common standards of her time. Again and again, she took on the patriarchs of the church in this regard, openly criticized them in sharp incendiary letters and even reprimanded King Barbarossa, to whom she regularly gave written lectures on the leadership of the empire.[1]

As a polymath, she also took up the cudgels for female writers with her books, specifically in literary areas such as worldview, spirituality, natural history and health teachings. Topics that women did not have to deal with in the opinion of medieval men's society.

For the modern women's movement, as well as for the female mystics of modernity, Hildegard is therefore more than a convent woman. She is a politician, women's rights activist, critic of religion and, last but not least, also a leading medical figure in the field of nutrition and health teachings.

---

[1] Bingen.de: https://www.bingen.de/tourismus/hildegard-von-bingen/leben-und-werk/ratgeberin-und-mahnerin/hildegard-und-friedrich-barbarossa

Especially in terms of nutrition, von Bingen did both impressive and fundamental work. Most of her instructions for healthy nutrition are still valid today and their effectiveness can now even be proven by corresponding study results.[2]

And Hildegard's recommendations are more relevant than ever. Many of her treatment measures are essentially based on a natural diet, which in many places corresponds amazingly precisely to the guidelines of modern nutrition and follows the millennia-old experience of our ancestors in terms of cultivation and health effects of traditional foods.

In this regard, von Bingen's convictions are fully in line with the current food trend, which is moving away from the unhealthy eating habits of our modern civilization and back to the origins of traditional national cuisine.

With her extremely well-founded knowledge of the effects of various foods and herbs, the nun Hildegard set fundamental standards for a health-promoting diet through conscious food choices during her lifetime. And even today, Hildegard von Bingen's nutritional philosophy serves as a reliable guide for all those who want to optimize their diet and thus contribute to maintaining or restoring their health.

Then as now, Hildegard's principles showed repeated successes in the therapy of diseases. Above all, she successfully treated digestive problems, gastrointestinal diseases, food allergies and metabolic disorders again and again thanks to nutrition plans individually tailored to her patients. Appropriate dishes were combined with exquisite herbs from her monastery garden, where she also grew most of the food herself.

Some crops and herb plants clearly had a higher value for the herbalist than others, and not without reason. According to Hildegard, certain crops have a particularly extensive health benefit. She also said that many cultivated plants, which today are only traded as conventional foods, are suitable for medicinal usage.

This is especially true for spelt, which has been proven to be one of Hildegard's favourites.[3] According to today's state of science, this is quite understandable, as spelt not only contains all the essential minerals and trace elements that our body needs every day. In addition, spelt also stands out for its, compared to other cereals, unusually high vitamin content and has some special active ingredients that make the plant almost a medicinal grain.

Another characteristic of nutritional herbs according to Hildegard is that the nun often relied on banal wild plants and weeds in floodplains and meadows, which today receive little attention as herbs. This applies, among other things, to the stinging nettle, which is more notorious as an inconvenient weed these days but was used by Hildegard in versatile a manner.

Whether as nettle tea or nettle soup – the herbal woman's nutritional applications of the plant were very comprehensive and ranged from the treatment of painful bladder infections to dehydration cures in the sense of metabolic cleansing. Hildegard also thought highly of more oriental to Far Eastern herbs.

---

[2] The Nutritional Therapy of Hildegard von Bingen by Wighard Strehlow: ISBN 978-3-426-65628-0
[3] St. Hildegard: https://www.st-hildegard.com/de/ernaehrung/dinkel/93-dinkel-die-15-eigenschaften.html

As a nun, Hildegard had access to the large archives of the church, in which literary treasures from all over the world were collected and translated into Latin, including numerous herbal books of Arabic and Asian origin.

For example, Hildegard knew a special recipe for garam masala consisting of nutmeg, coriander, cumin, cardamom, cloves, pepper, anise, fennel seeds, cinnamon and bay leaf.[4] And Hildegard was also no stranger to cooking with ginger, galangal and garlic, three relevant Far Eastern herbal roots with a strong antibiotic effect.

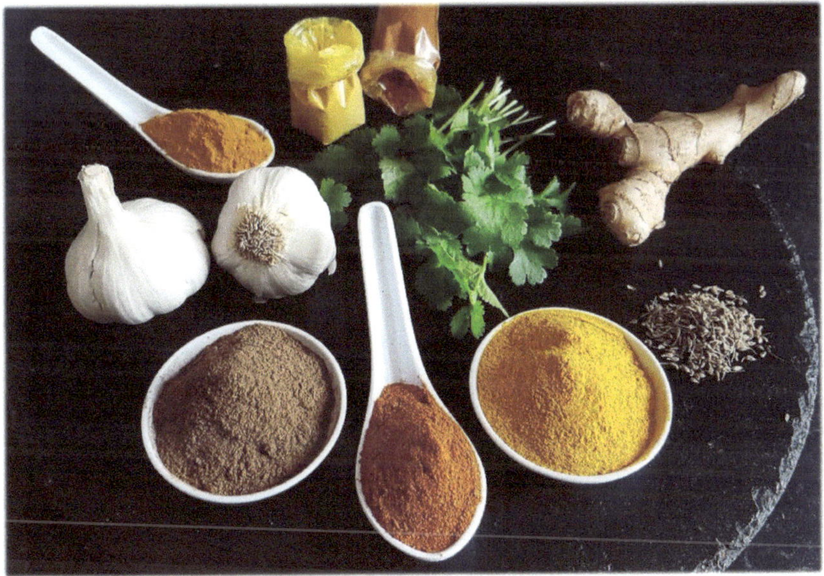

Already known in Hildegard's time: Ayurveda herbs

It can be said that Hildegard von Bingen's nutritional teachings have decisively shaped our current understanding of a healthy diet. The high importance she attributed to cereal plants such as spelt in the daily diet can be found today in the foundation of the current food pyramid, where grain and wholegrain products represent the most important food class, even before fruit and vegetables.

Her views on the importance of gently steaming or cooking vegetables for better nutrient preservation also hold true to this day. Not to be forgotten is her knowledge of numerous medicinal herbs, which has survived into modern times thanks to her first descriptions.

One can only speculate about what modern herbalism and nutrition would look like without the important cornerstones that Hildegard endowed thanks to writings such as

---

4 HVB healthy: https://hvb-gesund.de/wordpress/?page_id=10

her "Physica" or "Causae et Curae". At a time when more and more civilization diseases and allergies are triggered by wrong nutrition, her instructions are worth their weight in gold and are able to lead an ever larger number of people back onto the path of nutritional virtue.

Traditional cereals such as spelt are being rediscovered and the traditional way of eating, as it was still common for people in the Middle Ages and antiquity, is also finding more and more followers thanks to the in-depth knowledge of the health effects of food, as preached by Hildegard.

"For as the bellows kindle fire, and as wind and dew produce grasses, so also the juice of food and drink causes the blood, juice and flesh of man to arise and multiply"

Hildegard von Bingen

The Digestive Tract in the Focus of Health

When we talk about the digestive organs of humans, many people first think of the stomach and intestines. In fact, the two organ units form the core of the digestive system, whereby the food pulp in the stomach *(gaster)* is first coarsely decomposed. Of course, this does not happen immediately, but in spurts that are based on the interval-like release of stomach acid. The gradual decomposition of food in the stomach was also recognized by Hildegard. She wrote about the organ:

"[It] is created in the human body to absorb and digest all food. It is tough and rather wrinkled on the inside, so that it can retain the food for digestion and it is not digested too quickly, just as the mason works his stones in such a way that they accept and hold the mortar and (it) does not melt and fall to the ground."

After its coarse breakdown in the stomach, the food pulp finally reaches the small intestine *(intestinal tenue)*. This is where the actual nutrient extraction takes place, which gives the small intestine a particularly important role in metabolism. Above all, carbohydrates, fats and vitamins, as well as proteins are removed from the digested food pulp in the small intestine.

They are then passed on to the human bloodstream via the blood vessels of the small intestine before the food pulp is transferred to the large intestine *(Intestinum crassum)*. It is largely responsible for the drainage of the food pulp and the subsequent storage of the faeces, which are later excreted at regular intervals via the rectum.

The large intestine also includes the appendix *(Intestinum caecum),* which is sometimes quite inconspicuous. Supposedly inconspicuous, because contrary to the widespread assumption that the appendix is a rudimentary relic of human evolution that no longer has any special functions in the body, it is now known thanks to modern research that the caecum actually performs very important tasks in the area of immune defence.[5]

In the manner of the palatine tonsils, which take samples of food and cell residues from the oral cavity at regular intervals in order to have them examined for possible pathogens by the lymph nodes in the palate area, the lymphatic tissue of the appendix also seems to continuously monitor the immune status of the large intestine. In addition, enzymes necessary for digestion are produced in the appendix, which help the large intestine to break down stubborn dietary fats.

As a retreat for the intestinal bacteria, the appendix is also important with regard to the health-relevant intestinal flora *(intestinal microbiota)*. The term refers to the natural colonization of the gut by microorganisms that have entered into a natural symbiosis with the human body in the course of evolution. Modern molecular analyses have shown that the bacterial colonization of the intestinal flora alone results in a sum of 36,000 bacterial species, which on the one hand help to decompose the food pulp in the small

---

5 Science Daily: https://www.sciencedaily.com/releases/2017/01/170109162333.htm

and large intestines, but on the other hand also take on an immunological protective function within the intestinal flora.[6]

Again and again in the spotlight are the so-called lactic acid bacteria. As the name suggests, they produce a secretion called lactic acid in the intestine, which wraps around the intestinal mucous membranes like a protective film and thus protects the intestinal walls from attacks by potential pathogens. In addition, the intestinal bacteria themselves also actively help to fight pathogens, which makes them an important component of the adaptive immune defence.

All in all, it can be said that the intestine is essential for the production of nutrients as well as for the formation of secretions and the body's immune defences. Regarding secretion in the body's balance, the intestine provides the necessary nutrient building blocks for blood formation and the production of other body fluids such as mucus or digestive secretions.

Disorders in the area of intestinal function can therefore lead to serious problems in secretion and blood formation, which sometimes leads to serious illnesses. Hildegard's interpretation of secretion formation was, of course, somewhat more archaic in view of the state of research at the time, but testifies to quite logical and thus early scientific approaches:

"When man eats and drinks, a vital, rationally regulated attraction in man leads the taste, the finer juice, and the smell of the food and drink upwards to his brain, and warms it by filling his fine vessels. The other components of these foods and drinks, which enter the stomach, warm the heart, liver and lungs; they draw from this taste, the fine juice and the smell into their fine vessels, so that they are filled, warmed and nourished by it, as if a completely dried piece of intestine were placed in the water and it becomes soft, swells and fills up."

As a central organ complex of digestion, the importance of the stomach, large and small intestine within the body's own nutrient utilization is actually familiar to everyone. However, significantly more organs are involved in digestion than the gastrointestinal tract. For example, the liver *(Hepar)* is largely responsible for fat digestion. For this purpose, the organ produces the so-called bile juice, which flows through the ducts of the gallbladder *(vesica biliaris)* into the duodenum, the first section of the small intestine, where it helps to decompose fat molecules.

The ducts of the pancreas also open into the duodenum. It too produces digestive enzymes that help in the extraction of nutrients in the small intestine. And even the upper part of the urinary tract can be counted among the digestive organs.

In detail, this refers to the kidney *(Ren or Nephros).* Its widely branched system of renal corpuscles, the so-called nephron, not only filters metabolic waste products from the bloodstream, but also absorbs the last remnants of nutrients that can be used by the body from the primary urine before it drains into the urinary bladder as final urine via the ureters.

---

6 Nature Immunology: https://www.nature.com/articles/ni1079

It probably goes without saying that digestion is a highly complex bodily process, whose trouble-free functioning is indispensable for physical health. If there are functional disorders within the digestive organs, there is not only a risk of digestive problems such as constipation or diarrhoea.

Likewise, persistent digestive disorders lead to a long-term nutrient deficiency, which in turn promotes a variety of diseases. Metabolic and immune diseases in particular can always be associated with impaired digestion, whereby the entire body generally reacts adversely to inadequate nutrient absorption due to digestion.

In this context, malnutrition and lack of fluids play a central role in the development of digestive problems. If the daily requirement of nutrients and fluids is not sufficiently covered, this naturally also has harmful effects on the functionality and thus the health of organs, body tissues and even mental performance.

Conversely, a risky health status can also manifest itself through digestive problems. Stress and mental strain in particular often lead to corresponding complaints, which means that the digestive tract also acts as a warning system for inconsistencies in the body's routine.

Last but not least, as mentioned, essential parts of the immune system are part of the digestive system, too. Immune deficiencies and infections therefore have the habit of increasingly speaking out about gastrointestinal complaints. Hildegard explicitly underlines the importance of a regulated fluid intake as a guarantee for trouble-free digestion and writes the following in her "Causae et Curae":

"When man eats, he works when he eats like a mill when grinding. By working while eating, people become warm and dry inside. So he begins to dry up inside, and that is thirst. Then he has to drink something and eat again, and when he gets dry again from the heat while eating, he gets thirsty again, and then he has to drink again. This is how he must behave while eating, because if a person did not drink while eating, that is, when he consumes something, he would have mental and physical problems and would neither produce a good blood fluid nor have a good digestion."

Plant-based Nutrition according to Hildegard von Bingen

In view of the great influence that the digestive process has on physical health, it is all the more important to maintain a well-functioning digestion and to ensure an adequate supply of nutrients and fluids to the digestive organs. Plant-based foods in particular are coming to the fore in this regard, as they contain the most vitamins and minerals of all foods. At the same time, green foods also have a high water content, which improves the body's fluid balance in the long term.

Furthermore, plant-based foods are rich in fibre, which cannot be used by the body, but stimulates digestion and consequently benefits the cleansing of the gastrointestinal tract. In many cases, fruits, vegetables and the like even contain healing ingredients that make many a plant-based food a medicinal plant with superfood qualities. This is especially true for leafy vegetables and berries. Two food groups in which the transition from food to medicinal plant is almost fluid.

Hildegard von Bingen was no stranger to the essential contribution of a "green" diet to trouble-free digestion. This is hardly surprising, because she came into contact with the culture and preparation of plant-based foods at a very early age. Until her entry as an Oblate into the Rhineland-Palatinate monastery of Disibodenberg near Odernheim am Glan, she spent her childhood on her parents' manor in Bermersheim. The farm was the economic centre of the region and was therefore responsible for the cultivation of the surrounding fields and pastures.

It can be assumed that Hildegard not only spent a lot of time in nature and exploring the wild plant world at a young age but was also familiar with the traditional cultivation of crops and their use in the kitchen. Based on this background, the fact that her early childhood upbringing paved the way for the career of a nutrition-oriented healer, who often focused her treatment methods very specifically around a healthy nutritional concept, seems almost fateful. However, not everything that is celebrated as healthy today also corresponded to Hildegard's ideas of healthy nutrition.

For example, various crops, the daily consumption of which is highly recommended in modern times, were viewed rather critically by Hildegard regarding the actual health benefits. She also made strong distinctions in individual diets for sick patients and deliberately omitted supposedly healthy foods that tended to hinder recovery in the event of illness.

In return, an abundance of traditional fruit and vegetables, which hardly anyone remembers today, were part of the basic equipment of the Hildegard kitchen. Overall, however, Hildegard's dietary guidelines coincide strikingly with those of modern health experts and suggest that the healer had a comprehensive understanding of the functionality and interaction of herbal ingredients with the human organism.

Cereals and Nuts

Hildegard von Bingen was without doubt a great advocate of whole grain products. The grain cultivation of her parents, who as landlords filled the granaries of the rural population, may have contributed decisively to the conviction of the healer to regard grain products not only as a plant-based food, but also as a medically relevant nutritional measure. Accordingly, cereals and nut fruits were always on the menu of her patients, for example in the form of wholemeal bread, pasta or cereal porridge.

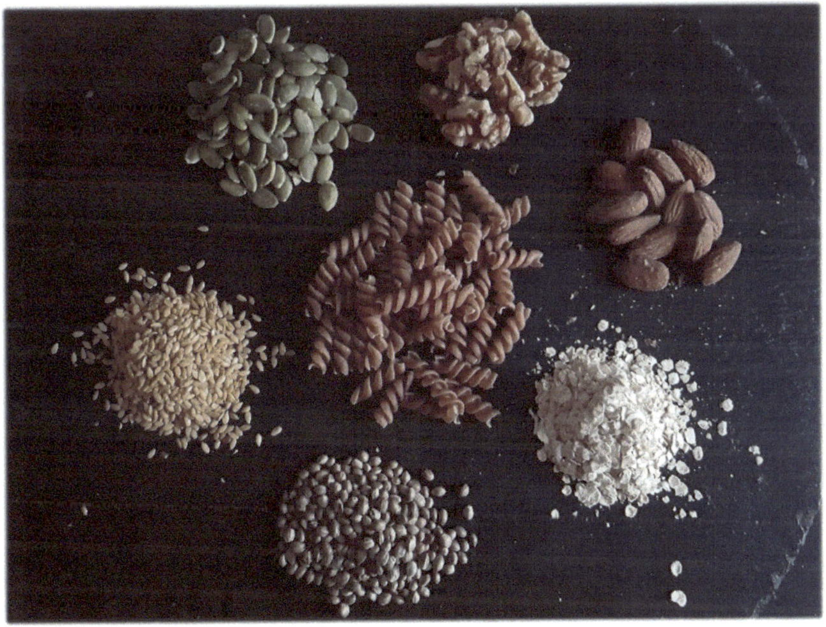

Products made from whole grains and nuts had a very special status for Hildegard.

Above all, Hildegard would not tolerate any bad word about her beloved spelt products, as spelt was by far her favourite grain. More than justified, because among all cereals, spelt is considered particularly healthy and incredibly undemanding in terms of cultivation conditions.

Spelt grain is exceptionally robust, which was a clear plus point by the standards of the time. Thanks to its excellent winter hardiness, it was very easy to grow even in the coldest regions of Northern and Central Europe, promising a good harvest.

In Germany, where a centuries-long cold period had just come to an end during Hildegard's time, frost-hardy spelt was probably the most important grain. It was the basis for the preparation of numerous foods and contributed to people's health to a considerable extent.

This is because spelt grain contains various health-relevant qualities. On the one hand, it is particularly easy to digest thanks to its delicate but fibre-rich peel, which relieves the stomach and intestines. Furthermore, spelt also contains many nutrients, sometimes up to twice as many as conventional grains.

"Spelt prepares good blood, strengthens muscle growth and the gift of cheerfulness [...]"

The exclusive nutrients in spelt are known to strengthen muscles, bones, teeth and fingernails. They also have a warming effect, stimulate the metabolism and promote blood circulation. Qualities that are more than desirable in the context of an illness-related recovery phase.

By stimulating the metabolism and blood circulation, medical compounds can be distributed much faster in the body, which accelerates the healing process. In addition, harmful pathogens can also be removed more quickly due to improved secretion and blood circulation. Spelt thus also serves to cleanse the metabolism.

Vitamins and minerals in spelt grain per 100 g	
Iron	4.17 mg
Potassium	385 mg
Calcium	38 mg
Copper	0.62 mg
Magnesium	2.90 mg
Zinc	3.40 mg
Vitamin B1	0.65 mg
Vitamin B2	0.23 mg

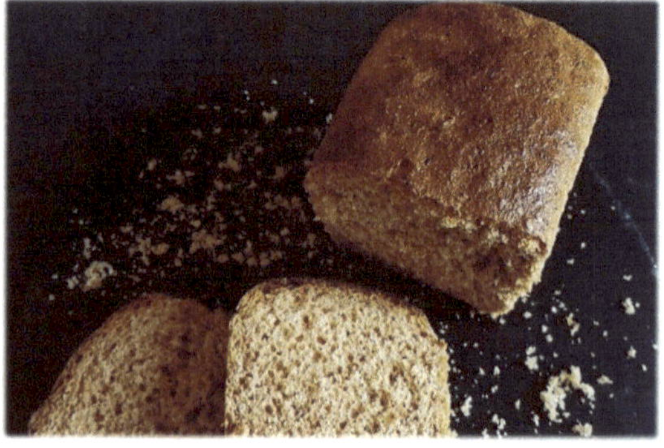

In addition to spelt, Hildegard von Bingen also relied on some other traditional grains and pseudo-grains. These include:

- Barley
- Unripe spelt grain
- Oats
- Hemp
- Millet
- Linseed
- Rye
- Wheat

Nut fruits, which are often very similar to cereals in terms of nutrient content, were also occasionally given health-promoting status by Hildegard. She classified almonds and walnuts as being just as muscle- and nerve-strengthening as spelt.

Almonds in particular also promised good help with liver complaints, metabolic disorders, kidney and urinary tract infections. In contrary, the abbess saw little benefit in hazelnuts, which, in her opinion, would not harm anyone, but otherwise had no appreciable healing effect either.

As with cereals, Hildegard also relied on varieties of nut fruits that were still considered traditional staple foods in her time but are now considered at best a popular snack or even a rare delicacy.

The best example of this are sweet chestnuts. Not to confuse with the non-edible conkers, chestnuts are almost exclusively available at Christmas markets these days. But the mother of all herb women even knew how to make remedies from the vitamin-rich fruits of the chestnut tree.

Hildegard recommended a mixture of 30 tablespoons of chestnut flour and 100 g of honey for mild liver ailments, whereby at least 2 teaspoons of sweet chestnut honey should be taken daily over a period of two months.

The chestnut flour is not only particularly rich in vitamin C and other important nutrients, but also gluten-free, which is why it also offers a wonderful alternative to regular flour for celiac patients.

Against gastrointestinal complaints, pancreas and severe liver and gall bladder diseases, Hildegard additionally prescribed a soup made from sweet chestnuts.

The antibacterial tannins, as well as the antioxidant flavonoids of chestnuts, were supposed to successfully relieve inflammation of the digestive tract. Chestnut saponins also have a mucus-busting effect and thus help to rehabilitate the gastrointestinal mucosa in the event of inflammation. Her soup recipe:

"If you have a stomachache, boil the fruit in water for a long time, crush it into a pulp and then mix in a bowl some spelt puree with the addition of liquorice powder and a little less angel sweet root powder, boil another puree from it and then eat it, and it will cleanse your stomach and make it warm and strong"

Wild Fruits and Berries

When it comes to the consumption of vegetables, Hildegard was primarily dependent on the regional fruit supply due to the time in which she lived. Exotic fruits such as citrus fruits or bananas rarely found their way into Germanic realms back in her days and when they did, they were extremely expensive.

Too expensive for a monastery that deliberately relied on a minimalist, if not spartan way of life. Instead, traditional fruit was often used in the Hildegard kitchen, which is (unfortunately) hardly to be found in the national cuisine today. We are talking about old fruit varieties such as rose hips, medlars or quinces. They are all full of vitamins and were once easy-to-cultivate wild fruits and an indispensable part of the home kitchen.

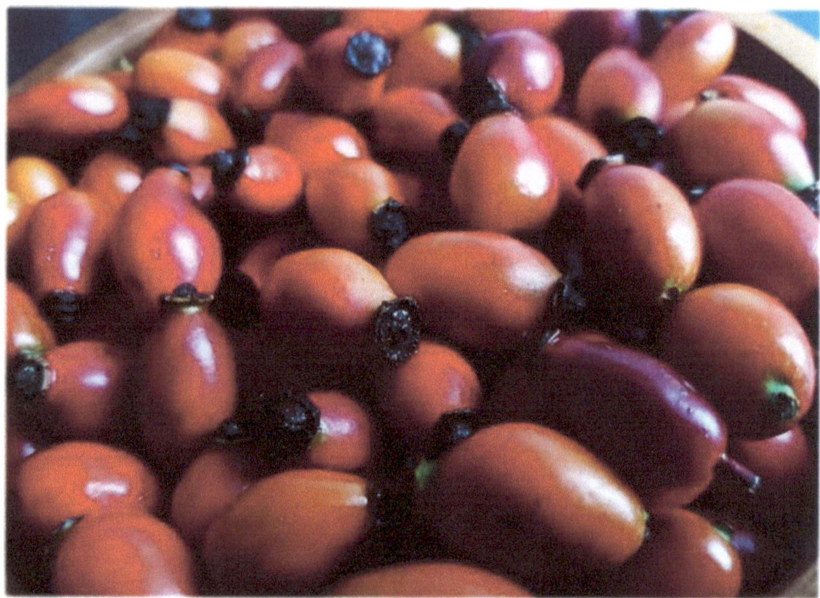

Domestic wild fruit such as rose hips were an important part of a healthy diet in the Middle Ages.

Today, unfortunately, rose hips and co. are usually only found as seasonal delicacies in experienced restaurants or orchards of tradition-conscious gardeners. It's a pity really, because they have been proven to be a recommended source of nutrients for gastrointestinal ailments and diarrhoea.

Of course, Hildegard von Bingen also relied on more common regional fruit varieties such as apples or pears, whose floury consistency once again facilitates digestion. In this respect, pome fruit clearly stands out from many other fruits that have a more fleshy interior. The same applies to cherries and although Hildegard emphasized that they are not particularly useful in terms of health, she stated that their consumption at least does not harm.

Important: While apples and cherries can also be eaten raw according to Hildegard von Bingen, she was strongly in favour of heating pears. Rose hips, medlars and quinces should also be warmed sufficiently before consumption and, if necessary, seasoned with brown sugar or honey, as the fruits are relatively inedible when raw.

Pectins are responsible for the firm yet incredibly floury flesh of apples, pears and cherries. A special type of polysaccharides that are still used today as a natural gelling agent to thicken jam, desserts and cake toppings. Compared to conventional table sugar, however, pectins are much healthier because more energy is needed to break them down in the digestive tract. Accordingly, intestinal activity is additionally stimulated during the digestion of pectins.

In addition to pome and stone fruits, the herbalist Hildegard already noticed local berries as carriers of extraordinary healing power. Today we know that this healing power is not only due to the high vitamin content of berries, but also to their plant pigments, the so-called flavonoids.

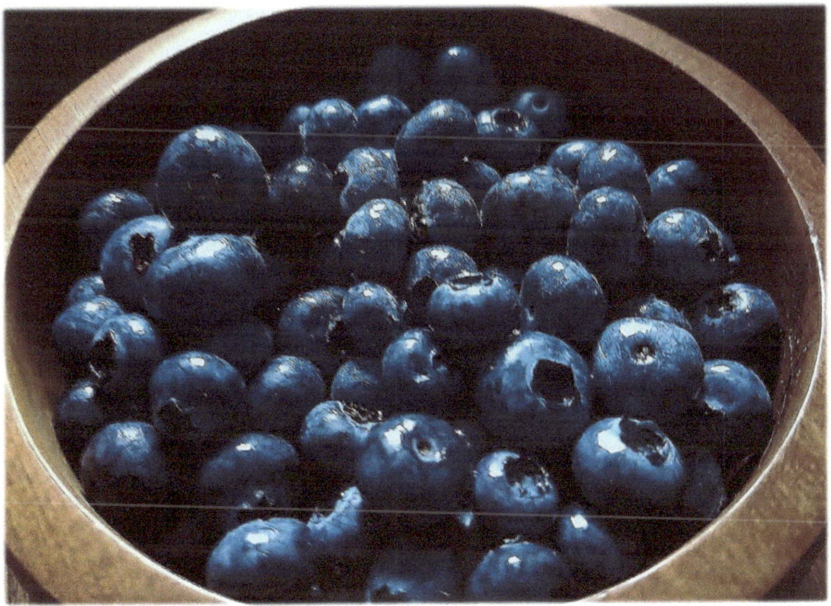

One of the best local antioxidant foods against digestive problems: blueberries and blueberries

The name of the flavonoids goes back to the Latin word *flavus* for "yellow", as the first plant pigments ever discovered were yellow-colouring substances of the dyer's oak. They were subsequently used to dye textiles and some are still in use for this purpose today.

Gradually, however, other plant pigments were discovered that colour orange, red, purple, blue and green in addition to yellow. In berries, red and blue to violet flavonoids are at work in that regard.

Of greatest medical importance are blue-violet to black-coloured flavonoids from the group of anthocyanins, which are particularly abundant in dark berry fruits.

Its special healing effect lies in an antioxidant, diuretic and anti-inflammatory effect, which is particularly popular with women to treat urinary tract infections. According to Hildegard von Bingen, the most important berry fruits in this section are:

- Blackberries
- Raspberries
- Currants
- Mulberries

Antioxidants have also been successful with heart and vascular diseases as well as digestive problems, as they rid the body of harmful waste products that impair metabolic activity, secretion and blood flow.

Vegetables and Salads

Hildegard's other all-rounders in the field of healing foods also include legumes of all kinds. Above all, beans, which she considered superior to peas and chickpeas in terms of health value and repeatedly used for gastrointestinal and kidney diseases.

The situation was similar with another favourite vegetable of the nun, fennel. To this day, it is considered one of the best herbal remedies for digestive problems and urinary tract diseases, as it has digestive and diuretic properties at the same time and such a gentle effect that it is even suitable for children and infants.

The third important vegetable pillar in the Hildegard kitchen are root vegetables. However, it is not the ever-popular carrots that set the tone in Hildegard's dietetics – carrots were not considered harmful by the healer, but also not particularly useful – but rather less popular beets and tubers such as:

- Garlic
- Parsnips
- Radish / Horseradish
- Beetroot
- Celery

According to Hildegard, they all contribute to a healthy flow of secretions in the digestive tract and regulate digestive processes, as they contain a high water content and an abundance of important minerals that are needed in the body to produce secretion. The abundant fibre contained in root vegetables also has a cleansing effect and stimulates intestinal peristalsis.

In addition, there are various leafy vegetables in the Hildegard kitchen, which also regulate digestion. Spinach is a wonderful all-rounder here, because on the one hand it is rich in water and thus provides large amounts of fluid, which is important for good digestion.

On the other hand, it has many vitamins and minerals, with the zinc in spinach in particular being considered to stimulate the metabolism. In addition, the fibre in spinach stimulates intestinal peristalsis, which also strengthens digestive function.

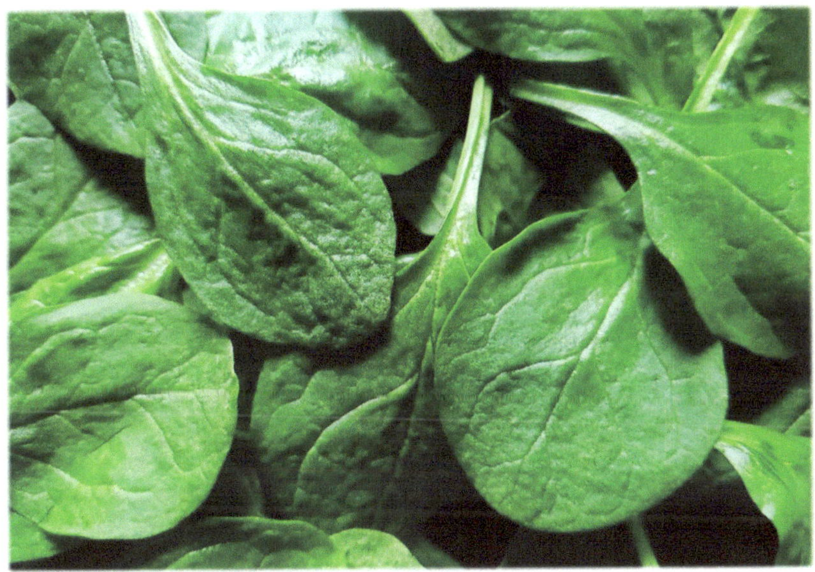

Among the most important leafy vegetables in Hildegard's kitchen: spinach

The situation is very similar to spinach with salad. However, in this case, Hildegard understands that a strong distinction must be made between individual types of lettuce. While she even gave seasoning tips for mild lettuce, for example – she suggested dressing the lettuce with garlic, dill and vinegar – she wrote about chicory, which is considered the parent genus of endive, radicchio and chicory:

"The chicory is warm and moist and symbolizes decency [...]
However, those who carry them with them incur the hatred of other people [...]"

In the language of a clergyman, it can be concluded that chicory should be treated with caution and used sparingly in the kitchen. The herb woman also looked at cabbage vegetables with mixed feelings:

„ [...] Your juice is of no use. They give rise to states of weakness because they injure weak intestines. Only healthy people who are not very fat can digest cabbage and cabbage through their strength. Cabbage is harmful to fat people because it bloats the meat even more. It is just as harmful to the sick. Cooked as a vegetable or with meat, cabbage increases the bad juices more than it diminishes them."

However, it should be said that cabbage vegetables and chicory are not harmful to health in principle. Especially in winter, cabbage varieties are an important source of nutrients as storage vegetables. However, in order to not overdo it with the flatulent vegetable, one should provide sufficient variety in the diet with other classic winter vegetables such as beets or potatoes.

Caution: Raw Food

Speaking of raw food, von Bingen was generally rather critical of such diets, which are celebrated today by staunch supporters as extremely healthy. Her argumentation for this, which was quite understandable from a conventional medical point of view, was that raw food means a massive additional effort for digestion when it comes to decomposing.

Hildegard sees the cause of this in a cold stomach, which, like a cold stove, cannot heat food afterwards. It therefore requires a warming energy supply from the outside that warms up the stomach in advance and thus "heats up" the digestive process, so to speak. In her opinion, only a warm stomach is able to "soften" the food pulp.

"When a person is sober, he should first eat food prepared from fruit and flour, because the food is dry and gives a person healthy strength. He should also eat a warm meal first, so that his stomach may be warm, and not cold food; because if he eats a cold food first, he makes his stomach cold, so that he can hardly get warm with hot food later. He should first eat a warm meal until his stomach is well warmed. When he then eats a cold dish, the heat that permeates his stomach copes with the subsequent cold in the food."

The convent nun is not entirely wrong with her statements. Since the food pulp has a relatively firm consistency when eating raw food compared to soft-cooked food, it takes longer to break down the food particles it contains. The food pulp thus lingers longer in the gastrointestinal tract, which causes more digestive gases to form and then causes flatulence and abdominal pain.

Raw grains, such as those found in muesli, also contain high amounts of phytin. The bioactive plant acid binds large amounts of minerals in cereals such as bran, which can therefore only be insufficiently absorbed by the body in a raw food diet.

Many vegetables, on the other hand, sometimes form toxic protective and bitter substances, which can only be neutralized by increased heat intake. The best example of this are nightshade and pumpkin plants. In this respect, the Pumpkin Family (Cucurbitaceae) not only have in common that they are related to the pumpkin.

Their plant parts also form so-called cucurbitacins in the same way. The name here is derived from the technical name of the Cucurbitaceae, which includes zucchini, cucumbers and melons in addition to pumpkins. Cucurbitacins are a subgroup of bitter substances that are supposed to protect the Cucurbitaceae against predators and fungal diseases.

The fact that plant toxins are also able to do something against the predator humans is proven by numerous food poisonings with a fatal course that occurred in the past after eating raw pumpkins.

As far as Nightshade Family *(Solanaceae)* are concerned, the consumption of raw potatoes in particular is not recommended. The tuber vegetable, which once came to Europe from America with other nightshade plants such as peppers or tomatoes, is known for its high content of the plant toxin solanine. It is very concentrated in most parts of the Solanaceae plant, which is why the plant family is considered particularly poisonous, except for its few edible representatives.

How deadly the consumption of nightshade plants can be is proven by patented poisonous plants such as belladonna or the nightshade that gives the plant family its name. In the potato tuber, the solanine is mainly concentrated on the root eyes, which develop after the germination of the tuber, as well as on green areas of unripe potatoes.

Since solanine is also heat-resistant, green and germinating potatoes should not be eaten raw or cooked. And even unripe tomatoes are dangerous. Already 100 g contain up to 32 mg of the toxic solanine, whereby 400 mg can already lead to death. So, one should only eat ripe nightshade vegetables.

A third group of plant-based foods that was problematic for Hildegard von Bingen were the species of the Leek Family *(Allioideae)*. With the exception of garlic, which she counted among the healing tuber vegetables, she had mixed feelings about leek vegetables such as onions. Under no circumstances should they be eaten raw, according to the advice of the herbalist and this not even as a finely chopped ingredient for salad dressings.

Onion is also not recommended for people who suffer from digestive problems. It especially "causes pain to stomach sufferers because it is moist," she writes. In fact, the high sulphur content of onion can lead to very painful flatulence and even cramps and colic in people who already suffer from a sensitive stomach.

With a healthy stomach, however, Hildegard seemed to have no objections to eating onions. What's more, cooked onions would even help people with fever, gout, heart and vascular diseases.

In the area of digestion, onions also support a healthy appetite as well as saliva and stomach secretion, which is consequently beneficial for digestion. Again, however, only if the onion has been sufficiently cooked beforehand and not eaten raw. The situation was completely different with the above-ground plant parts of the leek, which Hildegard counted among the so-called kitchen poisons.

Hildegard's Kitchen Poisons

Not only raw vegetables, but also various types of fruit and vegetables, which can be confidently consumed daily according to modern understanding, were anything but harmless according to Hildegard's understanding and were treated by her as kitchen poisons.

By this, she meant various plant foods that, if consumed too frequently, disrupt the flow of secretions in the digestive tract, excessively congest it or promote allergic reactions and skin rashes. Some examples of such herbal kitchen poisons are:

- Apricots
- Strawberries
- Peaches
- Plums
- Leek

In fact, at least for leeks, it can be proven that they stimulate the proliferation of leukocytes in the blood due to their high sulphur content. Which, in turn, can provoke excessive pus formation. An increased production of bile acid can be observed after eating plums, which can have a sensitive effect on the pH value of the digestive tract in the long run.

In the case of strawberries, the fact that the fruits grow dangerously close to the ground made things even more difficult in Hildegard's opinion. As a result, the fruits increasingly absorb harmful soil toxins and fungi, which subsequently promote the development of allergies and infections.

In the case of peaches, only special preparation, such as removing the skin, sufficient cooking or pickling in wine or vinegar, could neutralize the toxic components that promote allergies, according to Hildegard.

Medicinal Herbs for gastrointestinal Problems

As already shown, Hildegard von Bingen always placed a special focus on the gastrointestinal tract in her nutritional and herbal therapy. As is well known, this gut section also forms the core element of digestion and is sometimes particularly susceptible to complaints of health issues. That being said, it is not only local diseases that can severely affect the stomach and intestines.

Disease progression in adjacent organs as well as nervous and mental stress are also repeatedly noticeable through corresponding digestive problems in the gastrointestinal section. One of the most common non-specific symptoms here is loss of appetite.

Loss of Appetite

A lack of appetite is common not only in specific gastrointestinal diseases, but also in fever and infectious diseases. Eating disorders, food poisoning and depressive moods too are characterized by loss of appetite as a side effect.

In many cases, this is due to a nutrient deficiency – especially vitamin deficiency. Which occurs very easily in the context of an illness because the body consumes an above-average amount of nutrients for regeneration. Likewise, numerous medications and disease-related changes in the sense of taste tend to reduce appetite.

Nutrient deficiency as a cause of loss of appetite can often be regulated by the mere use of plant-based foods from the Hildegard kitchen. While fruit contributes plenty of vitamins to recovery, vegetables and grains provide valuable minerals to strengthen the metabolism and immune system. In addition, good will is often helpful. Although one shouldn't have to force themself to eat, knowing that your appetite will return faster if you give it a boost with taste stimuli can provide sufficient motivation to eat.

If the loss of appetite is particularly persistent, medicinal herbs are also recommended to increase the feeling of hunger. In this regard, Hildegard relied in particular on aromatic herbs such as Clary Sage *(Salvia sclarea).* Unlike its famous relative, the common sage, this sage species does not bloom blue, but white-pink and is also much spicier in its aroma.

The leaves of clary sage also differ significantly from those of its famous conspecific, which can sometimes help identify wild plants. While the latter is conspicuous by narrow, elongated-oval leaf lobes, the clary sage is characterized by much larger, more heart-shaped leaves, which are usually very felty.

Clary sage is also commonly known as Roman sage because its use has a long tradition especially in the Mediterranean region. Hildegard therefore owes her knowledge of the plant in part to ancient written sources from Roman-Greek antiquity. She liked to use the medicinal plant together with other appetizing herbs such as Pennyroyal *(Mentha pulegium)* and prepared a potion from them with a little honey and white wine to stimulate the feeling of hunger in order to treat not only loss of appetite but also digestive problems.

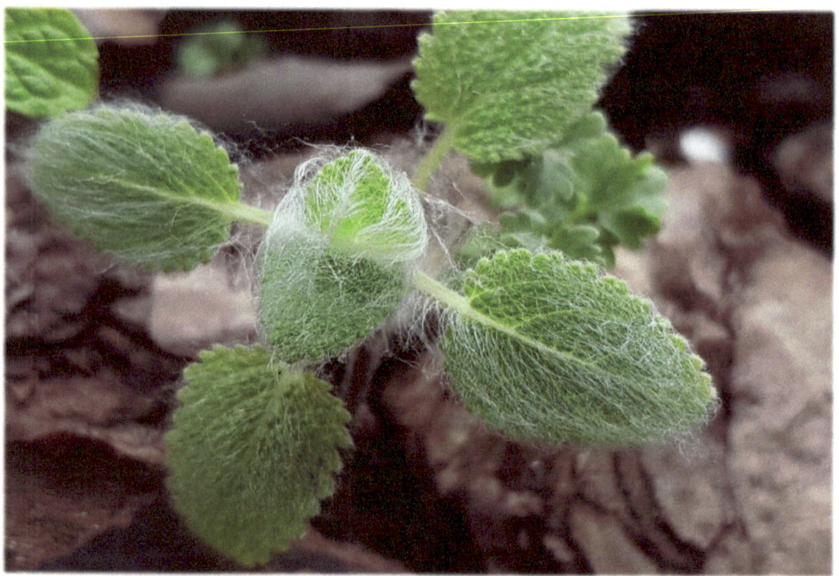

Clary Sage Elixir:	Put the leaf and seed herbs together with the wine and honey in a saucepan and let the whole thing boil for 3 to 5 minutes.
- 1 l white wine - 50 g honey *(skimmed)* - 10 g leaves of clary sage - 6 g leaves of pennyroyal - 2 g fennel seeds	Then strain the potion through a sieve. Taking 1 to 2 liqueur glasses of the elixir daily as an aperitif promotes the appetite. Drunk after lunch and dinner, the elixir also improves digestion.

Tip: *To store the elixir, it is important to fill it into a dark, airtight bottle to increase its shelf life. However, those who suffer from a weak stomach should only take the potion by the teaspoon.*

It is noticeable that the herbs used by Hildegard against loss of appetite are often also able to do something for digestive problems. Mother Nature obviously has a preference for the compact mode of action of her digestive herbs. This is especially true when it comes to the gastrointestinal tract.

Stomach Problems

Similar to loss of appetite, inflammation can sometimes have many different causes. Gastritis is the best example. Depending on the cause of the inflammation, a distinction can be made between up to 5 different gastritis variants, whereby in addition to infectious agents, autoimmune processes, chemical substances and even the body's own secretions in the form of stomach acid or bile can be the cause of the inflammation.

However, bacterial pathogens such as Helicobacter pylori are most often responsible for gastritis. These initially cause persistent irritation of the stomach mucous membranes until they finally become inflamed and subsequently begin to decompose. Since the mucous membranes of the stomach are very explicitly affected by the inflammation, the term gastritis is also often referred to as mucous stomach inflammation. Typical accompanying symptoms of gastritis are

⇨ Feelings of pressure in the stomach area

⇨ Stomach-ache

⇨ Heartburn

⇨ Digestive issues

If the inflammation is not treated promptly, it can even lead to stomach bleeding and, later on, dangerous degeneration of the gastric mucosa, which then results in a Stomach Ulcer (Ulcus ventriculi). The degeneration of the mucous membrane is much more dangerous than mere gastritis and increases the risk of stomach cancer in the long term.

The stomach pain that occurs with a stomach ulcer is particularly unbearable and usually reaches its peak immediately after eating food, when more stomach acid is released for digestion. Due to the inadequate mucosal protection caused by the disease, the aggressive acid can directly attack the stomach walls, which sometimes causes colic-like pain. Digestion itself can also suffer from this colic, so that a blockage of the stomach due to persistent cramps cannot be ruled out.

„[…] if you suffer from constipation in the stomach and abdomen, pulverize ginger and mix this powder with a little juice of ox tongue. And from this powder and bean flour he makes tartlets, and he bakes them in an oven whose fire heat has subsided somewhat. And so let him eat these tartlets often after eating and on an empty stomach, and it reduces the filth of the stomach and strengthens the person […]"

The Hildegard kitchen knows many different herbs for stomach diseases. Amazingly, the herbalist of the Middle Ages used various aromatic herbs for many of her recipes, which today are more likely to be attributed to the Far Eastern disciplines of Ayurveda and Traditional Chinese Medicine. Both Ginger (Zingiber officinale) and Galangal (Alpinia galanga), two root herbs that are classically attributed to Asian medicine, Hildegard knew how to use in a variety of ways. This is not without reason, because both ginger plants are considered exceptionally anti-inflammatory, antispasmodic and analgesic. In addition, they regulate the secretion of stomach acid and bile juice, which benefits digestion.

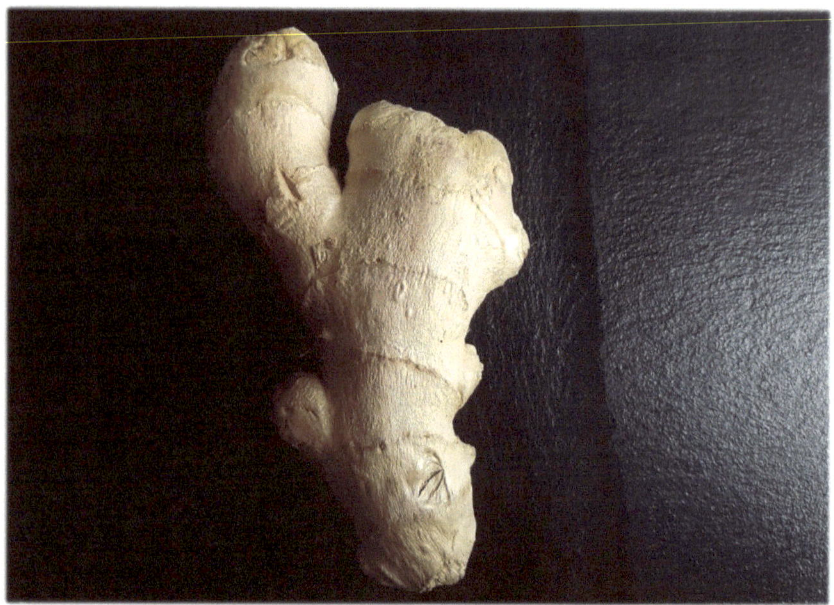

Ginger Mixed Powder:	The pre-dried root herbs are ground in a mortar into a fine powder.
- 20 g galangal root - 10 g ginger root - 5 g white turmeric root *In this mixed powder we find three ginger plants chosen by Hildegard, hence the name "ginger mixed powder".*	Alternatively, you can also buy galangal, ginger and turmeric pre-ground or pre-dried in the pharmacy or health food store. For the application, 1 to 3 pinches of the ginger mixing powder are then placed in a liqueur glass full of wine and drunk after eating and before sleeping.

***Tip:** By the way, a stomach-friendly wine can be made very easily from 2 to 3 teaspoons of laurels and 500 ml of red wine. Both boiled in the pot for about 3 minutes and then filtered, forms a wonderful basis for taking the ginger mixed powder.*

Hildegard's knowledge of Far Eastern medicinal herbs from the ginger family was most likely due to her access to the monastic herb archives. Medicinal herbal writings from all over the world were stored here and waited to be translated by the clergy into the church's Latin that was common at the time. Copies of exotic herbs often came from Greece or the Arab world, where Indian medicinal herbs were in use long before the beginning of the Middle Ages.

The nun knew how to use not only Asian herbs, but of course also banal native plants against stomach problems. Her use of of exquisite deciduous tree herbs such as the Sweet Chestnut *(Castanea sativa)* or the Field Elm *(Ulmus minor)* seems particularly interesting.

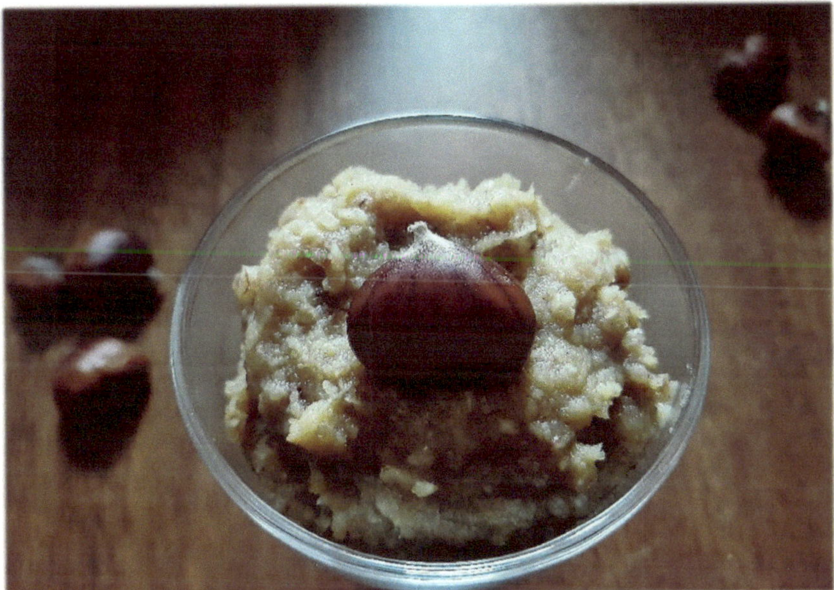

Chestnut Licorice Root Mixed Powder:	Elm bark porridge:
- 60 g liquorice root powder - 40 g of angel sweet powder - 1 tsp flour of sweet chestnut - 1 bowl of Habermus	Mix 2 teaspoons of elm bark powder with lukewarm water or milk until it has a mushy consistency. If taken a few teaspoons of it daily, the porridge can improve the mucous membrane protection of the stomach (e.g. for heartburn).

For stomach problems, take the elm bark porridge or 1 tsp of the mixed powder mixed in a bowl with Habermus daily for breakfast for 4 to 6 weeks.

The tree herbs mentioned are known for their rich content of mucilage, which is repeatedly used in medicine to treat inflamed mucous membranes. In addition, mucilage also alleviates the pain potential of mucosal inflammation, stomach pain and heartburn, as it has a calming and cooling effect.

Intestinal Diseases

The field of intestinal diseases and intestinal complaints is much more extensive than that of stomach diseases. Intestinal inflammation is an important group here, whereby a distinction must be made between different forms of intestinal inflammation depending on the location and clinical characteristics:

⇨ Inflammation of the duodenum (Duodenitis): An inflammation of the mucous membranes in the duodenum, which is often related to a previous gastritis or intestinal infection. Further conceivable causes are heavy alcohol consumption, certain medications (especially rheumatism drugs such as NSAIDs), nerve irritation and inflammatory diseases of neighbouring organs such as the gall bladder or pancreas.

⇨ Inflammation of the small intestine (Enteritis): It is usually caused by small intestinal infections due to bacteria such as Campylobacter, Clostridia, Escherichia coli, Salmonella, Shigella or Staphylococci, more rarely viruses such as adenoviruses and rota viruses or protozoa such as amoeba.

Aggressive radiation therapies in the context of cancer and intoxications such as those caused by food poisoning are also conceivable as triggers. A special form of inflammation of the small intestine is also the gastrointestinal inflammation known as stomach flu.

  ⬦ Gastrointestinal Inflammation (Gastroenteritis): A combined inflammation of gastritis and enteritis, in which bacterial pathogens can often be identified as triggers. In most cases, food poisoning, for example due to salmonella or a lack of food hygiene standards, are responsible for the causative infection.

⇨ Inflammation of the colon (Colitis): Similar to enteritis, infectious agents are the most common cause for colitis. In addition, there are radiation- and drug-associated forms of colitis. The latter often occur as a result of antibiotic treatment, which attacks the natural bacterial environment of the intestinal flora as well as bacterial pathogens. Additionally, there are three important chronic forms of intestinal inflammation

  ⬦ Colitis ulcerosa: A chronic inflammatory bowel disease limited to the mucous membranes of the colon that causes immense digestive problems for patients. The causes of ulcerative colitis are not fully understood yet, but experts suspect a hereditary tendency to inflammation as well as pathologically increased immune reactions behind the disease.

  ⬦ Morbus Crohn: Even though identical to ulcerative colitis in its suspected causes, Crohn's disease is also decidedly different from it when it comes to the extent of the inflammation. In addition to the large intestine, the small intestine, stomach and even the oesophagus can be affected. The assumption that Crohn's disease is an autoimmune disease has not yet been confirmed, but it is not unfounded.

↳ Diverticulitis: This inflammation manifests itself in the diverticula of the intestinal walls. These describe natural protrusions of the intestinal mucosa, which are actually benign and do not require any special treatment as long as they do not cause any symptoms. If there is an increased amount of diverticula in the colon, however, they are increasingly susceptible to inflammatory processes, which also promote colorectal cancer if left untreated.

⇨ Inflammation of the appendix (Appendicitis or Typhlitis): If appendicitis only affects the appendix of the organ, it is called appendicitis. It is repeatedly triggered by smaller foreign bodies such as cherry, melon or grape seeds, which stray into the appendix during digestion and thus lead to inflammatory irritation. In contrast, a combined inflammation of the appendix and the ascending colon is referred to as typhlitis. Their development is usually due to a reduced level of neutrophil granulocytes in the blood, as is the case during chemotherapy. If left untreated, appendicitis carries the risk of serious secondary diseases, including tissue necrosis, peritonitis and intestinal perforations.

Although so different in their severity, most intestinal inflammations show the same symptoms, namely inflammatory tissue irritation and complaints in the form of abdominal pain, flatulence, intestinal cramps, diarrhoea and constipation. In the case of intestinal inflammation, they often occur specifically after food intake or after the consumption of certain high-risk foods (e.g. spicy or acidic food) and severely affect the digestive tract through repeated disturbances of the functional process.

One of Hildegard's herbs par excellence for such digestive complaints was Fennel (Foeniculum vulgare), which is still used in many ways today. For centuries, it has been one of the most important herbs in digestive schnapps, which proves its healing properties for intestinal complaints.

Fennel has such a gentle effect that it is even well tolerated by children and infants. Even as a kitchen spice and traditional vegetable, fennel can be consumed daily without hesitation. His tea brew, as well as extracts of his seeds, should therefore not be missing in any kitchen.

"Even eaten raw, fennel does not hurt. However fennel is eaten, it makes people happy and gives them pleasant warmth and good sweat, and it causes good digestion. Its seed is also of a warm nature and useful for human health when it is added to other herbs in remedies. For he who eats fennel or its seed daily on an empty stomach reduces the foul mucus or putrefaction in it, and suppresses the foul smell of his breath."

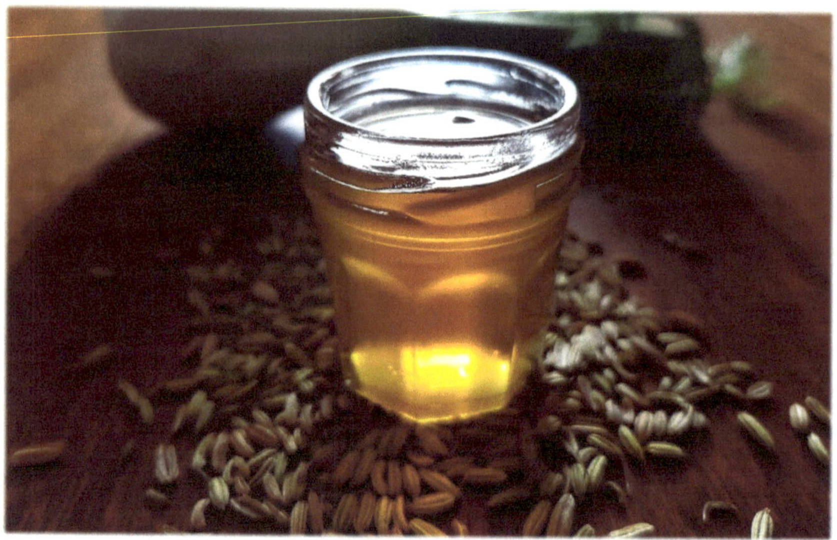

<table>
<tr><td>

<u>Fennel Mixed Powder:</u>

- 16 g fennel seeds

- 7 g anise seeds

- 5 g galangal powder

- 2 hawkweed powder

Crush the fennel and anise seeds in a mortar to a fine powder and then mix in galangal and hawkweed powder. Then put 2 to 3 knife tips of this mixed powder in a liqueur glass full of warm wine and then drink it daily after lunch.

</td><td>

<u>Mother Cumin Mixed Powder:</u>

- 36 g cumin seeds

- 4 g white peppercorns

Crushing the seeds of the mother cumin with the grains of white pepper into powder is often used to make "diarrhoea egg" according to the old model. To do this, mix a teaspoon of the mixed powder with six egg yolks, spread on a baking tray and bake dry at 100 °C for about 30 to 40 minutes. Then scrape the mixture from the bleak and serve the egg flakes with spelt bread.

</td></tr>
</table>

The secret of fennel lies in the special composition of its ingredients, which contain several components from essential oils and digestive flavonoids to minerals and vitamins from almost every medically valuable plant substance group.

Fennel is often mixed with Anise *(Pimpinella anisum)*, which, like fennel, belongs to the umbelliferous family and is very similar to it in terms of ingredient composition as well as aroma and effect.

In general, Hildegard von Bingen preferred to use herbs and spices from the ranks of the umbelliferous plants to treat intestinal complaints. As is so often the case, this is not without reason, because the aromatic herbs among the umbelliferous plants have in common that they are bursting with bitter substances. Behind this effect are bitter-tasting plant substances that are known to stimulate the secretion of digestive juices. Herbal and stomach bitters did not get their name by chance.

Cumin (*Cuminum cyminum*) also lives up to the reputation of bitter umbelliferous plants here. Another classic kitchen spice with a digestive effect, which, like its counterparts anise and fennel, can be found in many a herbal bitter. Cumin, also known as comyn or cymen in ancient times, yet again shows how familiar Hildegard was with oriental herbs. Because the spice is considered a cornerstone of Indian cuisine and consequently also has its place in the Indian healing art of Ayurveda.

The use of cumin mixed powder together with egg flakes and spelt bread furthermore underlines the importance of combining therapeutic measures within the Hildegard kitchen, which consist of herbs, spices and healthy nutrition.

Once again, Hildegard's grain products should be mentioned at this point. Spelt (*Triticum aestivum subsp. spelta*), formerly known as Dinkel wheat or hulled wheat, although Hildegard's favourite grain was by no means the only grain variant with a health-relevant effect that was used therapeutically.

Two other grains that promote digestion were also of great importance to her, namely Linseed (*Linum utisatissimum*) and Blond Plantain (*Plantago ovata*). Similar to sweet chestnut and elm bark, they contain valuable mucilage that wraps around the intestinal mucous membranes like a protective film and thus relieves inflammation and pain.

Often it is enough to sprinkle a heaped teaspoon of the easily swelling cereal seeds over the still warm food to elicit their mucilage. But if you want to be on the safe side, you can let them soak in water, milk or even natural yoghurt in advance. Milk and yoghurt also provide important lactic acid bacteria, which help to renovate the intestinal flora and thus further strengthen the weakened intestinal tract.

The herbal remedies mentioned above also help with another intestinal disease, which is all too often confused with intestinal inflammation due to its almost identical symptoms. We are talking about Irritable Bowel Syndrome.

Although it can certainly occur as a result of a corresponding inflammation and in particular persistent gastroenteritis, the exact causes of irritable bowel syndrome are still unclear. However, where opinions differ in conventional medical research on stress and hereditary causes, Hildegard cuisine has once again known advice for centuries.

The umbelliferous plants, which can confidently be described as explicit intestinal herbs in the Hildegard kitchen, are joined here by Coriander (*Coriandrum sativum*). From the ginger family, Hildegard recommends not only ginger itself but also the Mediterranean Cardamom (*Elettaria cardamomum*) against irritated intestines.

The herbs are widely used in Indian cuisine, which once again shows the knowledge of the clergy about the healing herbal treasures of the Orient. And even the unmistakably aromatic-spicy bark on the famous Cinnamon Tree (*Cinnamomum verum*) seems to have a calming effect on irritable bowel syndrome, according to her knowledge.

The herbs mentioned are just as effective for intestinal complaints such as diarrhoea or constipation, which is why they make for a good ingredient in any digestive tea. Together with gentle abdominal massages to relieve the intestines and light physical activity such as a long walk, digestion can quickly find its way back into balance.

Medicinal Herbs for Gallbladder Disorders and Liver Problems

The gallbladder and liver form an anatomical unit within the digestive complex. After all, secretions and nutrients are constantly exchanged between the two organs, including fatty acids, proteins, enzymes and blood pigments. Diseases of one of the two organs therefore affect the adjacent organ quite quickly, unless appropriate treatment is given.

Bilious Complaints

Bile problems already arise when the bile produced in the liver is prevented from passing through the bile duct. This can occur, among other things, due to Gallstone Disease (Cholelitiasis). Gallstones, known as coleliths, are always formed when crystalline deficits of bile occur in the gallbladder.

In addition to bile acid, bile consists mainly of cholesterol, protein and the bile pigments bilirubin and biliverdin, with cholesterol stones at about 80 percent being the most common gallstone variants and bilirubin stones being less common at about 20 percent.

Gallstones sometimes grow very slowly over a period of several years. They do not always immediately cause corresponding symptoms. Only when the stones have reached a certain size and repeatedly bump against the gallbladder walls does a gradually recurring and extremely painful colic set in.

In many cases, this persistent irritation of the bile walls also causes Gallbladder Inflammation (Cholecystitis). In addition, there is a risk that the stones will migrate into the bile ducts, which not only promotes more severe pain, but also stenosis in the area.

With such occlusions, the bile can no longer drain or only flow insufficiently, which leads to a Stasis Bladder (Gallbladder hydrops) in the further course. For digestion, this means that less and less bile enters the small intestine, which in turn massively impairs fat digestion. Digestive problems such as heartburn or flatulence therefore cannot be ruled out as secondary complaints.

If the bilirubin metabolism is permanently disturbed in the context of a biliary disease, it can lead to an increased concentration of the yellow bile pigment in the blood. The result is usually a pronounced Jaundice (Ikterus), which can also be caused by severe liver diseases. Signs of jaundice are clear yellowing of the skin, mucous membranes, and the sclera of the eyes.

"Whoever has jaundice, let him grind the saxifrage seed into wine and leave it for an hour. He often drinks it after eating, and the jaundice in him is extinguished, because it is sometimes triggered by an overflow of bile and something like this can often lead to hardening in the form of a stone."

Needless to say, treatment options for gallstones were very limited in the Middle Ages. The surgical removal of the stones was still completely unknown at that time, which is why the primary focus at that time was on the elimination or dissolution of the bile concretions by natural remedies.

A medicinal herb that even owes its name to its good effect against stone ailments of all kinds is a herb whose Latin name literally mean "stonebreak", better known as Saxifrage *(Saxifraga granulata).* Because both in its rocky locations in the wild and in the human organism, this medicinal herb breaks through stony obstacles without any effort.

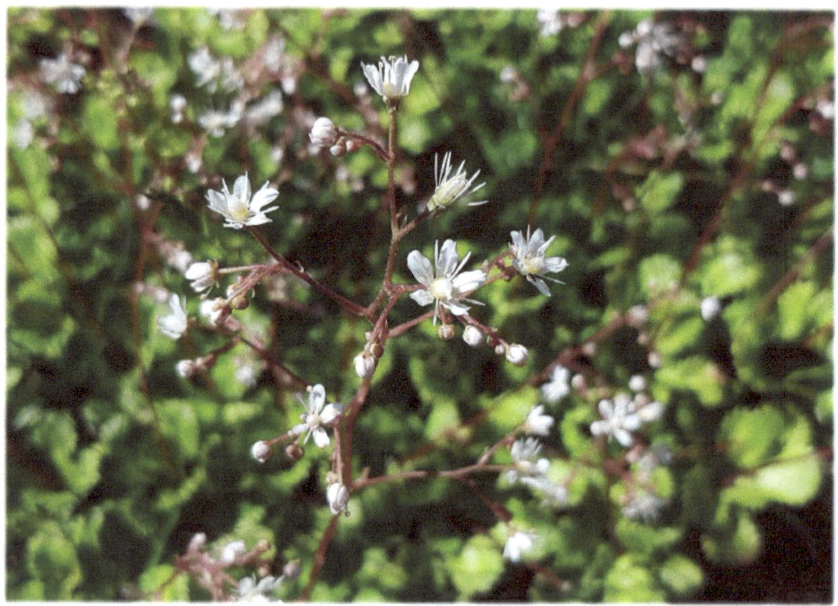

Sametic Seed Water:	Sametic wine:
- 2 g saxifrage seeds - 100 ml water	- 10 g saxifrage seeds - 1 l red wine
In the case of gallstones or gallstones, crush 2 g of saxifrage seeds in a mortar to a fine powder. Put a 1/2 pinch of it in a glass of water and drink it daily after eating, it is able to dissolve smaller gallstones.	The saxifrage seeds are soaked in 1 litre of red wine for about 60 minutes. After straining the seeds, 1 liqueur glass of saxifrage wine is drunk three times a day after eating if there is biliary disease.

The most important ingredients of saxifrage include tannins and bitters. Two plant substances that are known to have an incredibly stimulating effect on metabolism and digestion.

They also have anti-inflammatory and germicidal properties, which can be a valuable support for both biliary and liver inflammation. The astringent effect of saxifrage also ensures improved blood flow, which means that bilirubin residues in the blood can be removed more quickly.

Liver Problems

Bilirubin and biliverdin are degradation products of the red blood pigment haemoglobin, which is regularly broken down in the liver and replaced by fresh haemoglobin after a circulation period in the bloodstream of a maximum of 120 days.

In the aforementioned degradation process, the green biliverdin forms the precursor to the yellowish bilirubin. If there are complications in the liver's breakdown of haemoglobin, this not only has an impact on the production of bile.

Likewise, disorders in haemoglobin degradation promote serious liver damage. They usually begin with an increased storage of dietary fats in the liver tissue. In the long term, the consequence is a so-called Fatty Liver *(Steatosis hepatis).* A disease that can also occur after many years of malnutrition due to high-fat foods and often occurs in this context as a side effect of obesity.

Fatty liver is particularly dangerous for the functionality of the liver cells, which at some point become so overloaded with fatty acids due to the disease that they can no longer perform their blood-purifying task. Very similar damage to the liver cells is also caused by excessive alcohol, medication or drug consumption, which subsequently provokes downright liver poisoning.

Other conceivable triggers include liver infections and injuries to the liver. Regardless of the cause, damaged liver cells sooner or later inevitably lead to the development of Liver Inflammation *(Hepatitis).* As a secondary inflammation, this can also occur in the course of gallbladder inflammation. In general, inflammatory processes in the digestive tract tend to spread after a while of missing therapy. This is all the more the case if an infection is involved in the inflammation.

Therefore, if it comes to phytotherapy, herbs are in demand that relieve the liver, gall bladder and, if necessary, the gastrointestinal tract in the event of existing inflammation and reduce the risk of further secondary inflammation in adjacent organs.

A special recommendation of Hildegard in this regard is another long-forgotten traditional herb: the Common Agrimony *(Agrimonia eupatoria)* also known as Church Steeples. Once highly valued as an important anti-inflammatory and digestive medicinal plant, which was very well known even in North Africa and Asia, many people today do not even know the agrimony by name. And this despite the fact that its ingredients are still extremely relevant medically.

From rare tannins such as corilagin to tried-and-tested flavonoids such as apigenin and quercetin to high-quality plant acids such as silica, Agrimonia eupatoria doesn't lack any of the mentioned medicinal ingredients.

The holistic effect of agrimony on the entire digestive tract also includes gallbladder and liver protective aspects. There are even sources that report the effectiveness of Agrimony in acute liver failure. The best form of administration is as a tea herb in combination with other liver herbs.

<u>Tea blend with agrimony as liver herb:</u>

A mixture of herbs is prepared, which consists of 2 parts agrimony and 1 part each of dandelion, milk thistle, wormwood, chicory and calamus root. Take one teaspoon per cup of this tea mixture and add it to 250 ml of boiling water. After a brewing time of about 10 minutes, the tea herbs are strained and the tea is drunk in small sips. For 2 to 3 weeks, you can prepare up to 3 cups a day before a two-week break in use.

What is particularly dangerous about hepatitis is that it can cause much greater liver damage without suitable countermeasures. In the worst case, Liver Cirrhosis *(Kirrosis)* occurs, causing a gradual destruction of liver tissue.

The affected tissue can no longer regenerate at a sufficient pace due to an existing liver disease. Instead, more excess connective tissue forms in weakened sections of the liver tissue, which impairs blood flow to the organ and also seriously disrupts bile production.

Accompanying symptoms such as severe pain, inflammation-related mucus and even suppuration in the liver can no longer be ruled out in liver cirrhosis, which marks the dangerous final stage of many liver diseases. Liver failure is now an omnipresent danger to the patient's health and life. It is therefore important to relieve the liver as quickly as possible through in-depth nutritional measures and liver therapeutics.

Hildegard still knew what to do even against such serious conditions. She relied on an old fern plant, namely the Hart's tongue fern *(Asplenium scolopendrium).* Her hart's tongue elixir made from the herb is world-famous and still offered to liver patients in pharmacies today as a medicinal herbal liver therapeutic.

However, it should be mentioned that such treatments are not to be passed as an isolated measure in the case of severe liver damage. A well-founded medical treatment is without options here and can only be accompanied by medicinal herbs in a supportive way. This though in very reliable a manner.

"The hart's tongue helps the liver, the lungs and with painful intestinal complaints. [...] The hart's tongue elixir helps the liver, cleanses the lungs and heals the painful intestinal ailments, eliminates internal suppuration and mucus. [...] Drink it often before and after eating."

In the past, hart's tongue has been used again and again against a wide variety of diseases. Applications are known in pulmonology, urology, exhaustion and the treatment of sexual, glandular and gastrointestinal diseases.

Besides Hildegard von Bingen, other well-known healers such as Dioscorides, Pliny, Theophrastus, Hieronymus Bock or Otto Brunfels also mention it in this regard. They show that the healing effect of the hart's tongue fern has always been reassessed over the centuries and found to be significant. Overall, it is a proven medicinal herb whose long history of use confirms its good effects.

As a liver therapeutic, Asplenium scolopendrium helps the organ to break down substances through its polysaccharides that stimulate the immune and metabolic system on the one hand. At the same time, those polysaccharides also act as mucilage, which has a calming effect on the irritated tissue in the case of liver pain.

Last but not least, hart's tongue also contains tannins and antioxidants that act very specifically against inflammation and organ waste products. A plagued liver is therefore done something good in several ways by means of a hart's tongue elixir. Read Hildegard's original recipe for making the famous deer tongue elixir below.

Hart's Tongue Elixir: - 50 g flour - 20 g of deer's tongue fern - 10 g cinnamon bark - 1 g pepper - 1/2 l red wine	"The hirtzunge [hart's tongue] is warm and good for the liver, lungs and aching intestines. Boil them strongly in wine, add pure flour, then let it boil again, then powder long pepper and twice as much cynamomum [cinnamon] and let the milk boil again with the wine, press it through a cloth and make a luterdranck and drink it often sober as after breakfast."

Tip: A corresponding deer tongue cure is nowadays scheduled for 4 to 6 weeks of use, with a liqueur glass of the elixir to be taken 3 times a day after a meal in the first week. In the following weeks, a liqueur glass is served before and after the meal.

Medicinal Herbs for Urinary Tract Diseases

It can probably be rightly said that Hildegard von Bingen was also a gynaecologist. For herself, as well as for her nuns and the women from the surrounding estates of her monastery at Disibodenberg and later also around her monastery at Rupertsberg.

The latter was later founded by Hildegard herself and served as a pure nunnery, which may have directed her medical focus even more towards classic women's ailments. In addition to menstrual problems and obstetrics, urinary tract diseases were most likely the most common field of treatment in this context.

Bladder Diseases

The third organ complex in the digestive tract in addition to the gastrointestinal tract and the liver-gallbladder tract is the kidney-bladder tract. Ascending inflammation is a special complication here that especially women often have to deal with. Bladder Infection *(Cystitis)* in particular is often a recurring problem for the female sex. The reason for this is the woman's shortened urethra, which has a dangerously inviting effect on infectious agents.

Even the wrong wiping technique when going to the toilet can contribute to the development of cystitis. Besides, a lack of hygiene of women or men during or after the sexual act are among the most common causes for cystitis. The germs then rise relatively quickly to the urinary bladder and the typical accompanying symptoms feared by women develop in the form of a constant urge to urinate, unbearable pain when urinating and, in worst case, blood and pus admixtures in the urine.

There are a variety of helpful herbs against cystitis, such as chokeberry, bearberry, birch or Nettle *(Urtica dioica).* The latter is also a herb from the Hildegard kitchen and often is far too rarely valued as a medicinal herb, even though it is one of the best bladder herbs ever. Notorious as am unwelcome weed among gardeners due to its uncontrolled and fast-growing nature, nettles do not exactly enjoy the best reputation these days.

Gynaecology however has known how to use this herb successfully as a diuretic and anti-inflammatory herb since ancient times. It can be bought as a dried herb in almost any pharmacy and, as a medicinal herbal ingredient, can sometimes also be found in numerous natural remedies for cystitis. In addition to the nettle, Hildegard also recommended the following herbs against the number one women's disease:

- Field horsetail *(Equisetum arvense)*

- Marshmallow *(Althaea officinalis)*

- Goldenrod *(Solidago virgaurea)*

- Couch Grass *(Elymus repens)*

Ideally, the herbs are used for a diuretic and antibacterial tea blend that provides the body with additional fluid reserves at the same time. In this way, the urinary tract is sufficiently flushed in the event of illness and infectious agents are flushed out.

However, in order to prevent the body from drying out, only part of the tea mixture should consist of said herbs, especially in the case of goldenrod and couch grass. The medicinal plants are highly dehydrating, which can put an extreme strain on the body's fluid balance when used for several days.

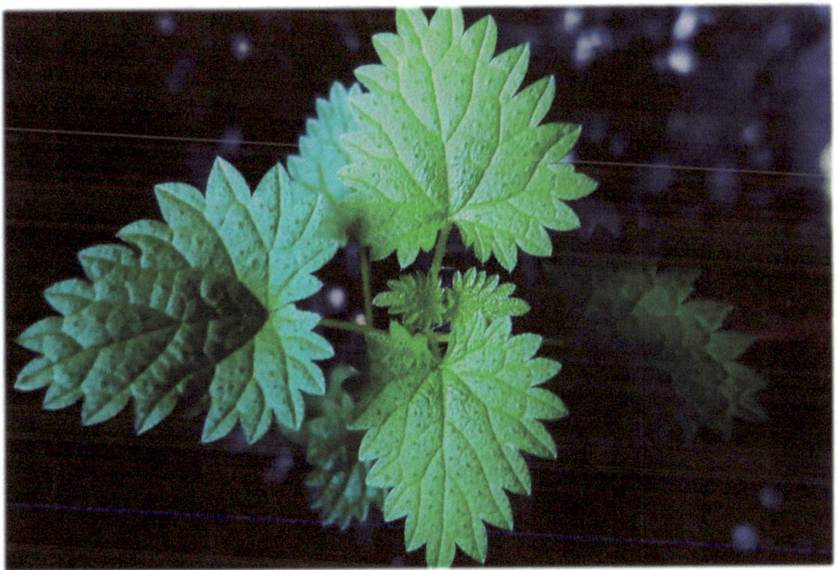

Tea made from bladder herbs:	Pour 500 ml of water over the tea herbs and let the decoction steep for about 5 minutes before filtering the herbs. Patients should drink 4 to 5 pots of this tea daily until the bladder infection subsides.
- 30 g field horsetail - 30 g nettle - 30 g marshmallow - 30 g goldenrod - 30 g couch grass	Acidic foods should be avoided in order to keep the pH value of the urine in the alkaline range and thus prevent unnecessary pain when urinating.

In addition, barley water and various berry juices can also be used. There are various berry fruits here, which have a particularly high content of antioxidant flavonoids from the group of anthocyanins and show a disinfecting and diuretic effect on the bladder and ureters in a similar way as corresponding leafy herbs.

This is especially true for dark berries, as they have the highest concentration of anthocyanins. In addition, the berries contain a wealth of vitamins that additionally strengthen the immune system and help it fight the infectious agents. The most important berry herbs for urinary tract diseases are:

- Black Chokeberry *(Aronia melanocarpa)*

- Blackberry *(Rubus sect. rubus)*

- Cranberry *(Vaccinum macrocarpon)*

- Blueberry *(Vaccinium myrtillus)*

All the herbs mentioned also help well against Bladder Stones *(Urolites)*, which are generally much more painful than urinary tract infections, but otherwise stand out due to a similar symptom. Diseases of the kidneys, into which initial bladder infections are only too happy to ascend if not treated, sometimes react very positively to conventional bladder herbs, too.

Kidney Diseases

Once pathogens have spread from a local urinary tract infection to the kidney, they usually immediately trigger a secondary inflammation in the form of Kidney Inflammation *(Nephritis)*. This is a dangerous development that inevitably threatens the functionality of the kidneys and is not to be trifled with, as it carries the risk of lifelong kidney insufficiency or even kidney failure. The intake of urinary tract herbs can therefore only offer supportive help for nephritis. In any case, comprehensive antibiotic therapy should also be given to avoid chronic courses.

Another kidney disease that is less associated with inflammation but with all the more severe pain symptoms are Kidney Stones *(nNeprolites)*. These are urinary concretions that are caused by crystalline precipitation of the urine and indicate a disturbed metabolism or an incorrect diet. Typical causes are, for example, metabolic diseases such as gout or diabetes as well as a diet of too many dairy products or foods rich in oxalic acid or purine.

In the kidneys, said causes then trigger a disturbed absorption of nutrients during urine formation. Which changes the material composition of the urine in such a way that it contains too many solids that then contribute to urine crystallization. Gout, diabetes and a diet rich in purines additionally often lead to the fall out of uric acid crystals.

Dairy products, on the other hand, promote the formation of calcium crystals and foods such as chicory, cabbage vegetables or rhubarb, which contain a lot of oxalic acid, can in turn provoke oxalate stones. In Hildegard's time, as with gallstones, the treatment of kidney stones and kidney semolina relied on medicinally active herb ingredients, which were able to dissolve the stone concrements and/or stimulate the flushing of the kidneys.

In addition to bladder and kidney herbs such as couch grass or marshmallow, Hildegard also knew very explicit kidney stone herbs, e.g. Oregano *(Origanum vulgare)*. A Mediterranean herb that is actually better known as a kitchen spice. In fact though, oregano also contains a wealth of disinfectant, diuretic and digestive ingredients that predestine the herb for use in gastrointestinal complaints and kidney diseases.

Oregano, together with marjoram, belongs to the genus Origanum and was also better known under the name "Dost" in the German Middle Ages. It was already used by the forefather of medicine, Hippocrates of Kos, as a medicinal herb to induce birth, which proves the long history of oregano as a medicinal plant. In the Middle Ages, the good effect of the herb against urinary tract diseases was also recognized, which is largely due to the bitter substances within the herb.

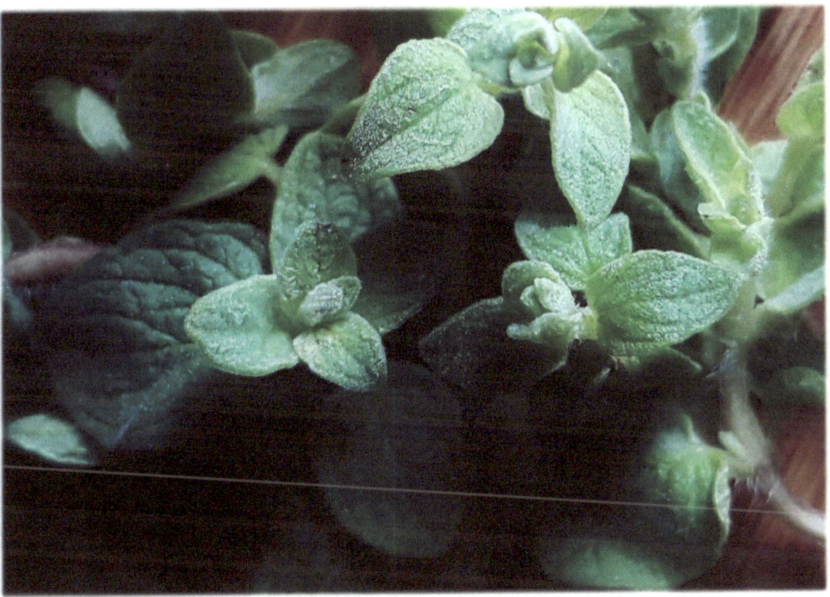

Tea against kidney stones:	The herbs are mixed together as usual and boiled with 500 ml of water to make a tea brew. The corn beard here is the hairy style of the corn cob, which is finely chopped for the preparation of the tea.
- 60 g oregano - 60 g marshmallow - 30 g glasswort - 30 g gingerwort - 30 g corn beard - 30 g of couch grass	Overall, Hildegard recommends drinking 2 to 3 litres of fluid in the urinary tract if you have a stone condition in the urinary tract, 1/2 litre of it in the evening and a total of enough to excrete at least 1/2 litre of urine per 24 hours.

Three other of Hildegard's kidney herbs stand out from the recipe above, because they are hardly used as such today. We are talking about:

- Upright Glasswort *(Parietaria officinalis)*

- Bedstraw (*Galium aparine)*

- Cornbeard *(Zea mays)*

Similar to the bladder herbs, the herbalist prepared a tea decoction from these medicinal plants, which she regularly prescribed to her patients to get rid of the urinary stones. An appropriate diet, which avoided critical foods that could contribute to further stone formation, was most likely the second pillar of Hildegard therapy against stone disease.

For Hildegard von Bingen, the preparation of herbal formulations for the medicinal treatment of digestive problems and diseases of the digestive tract was always accompanied by a nutritional guideline tailored to the special needs of her patients.

Depending on which foods could lead to complications in therapy, they were excluded from the diet plan and instead cereals, fruits and vegetables that had naturally healing properties were prescribed. In addition, the healer saw a healthy diet as indispensable in principle when it came to avoiding diseases.

From today's perspective, she was already spot on in the early Middle Ages. As doctors and nutrition experts now know, numerous diseases of the digestive tract stem from an unhealthy diet, which is particularly typical of the fast-paced society of the modern age. Old traditional foods are forgotten, as are traditional herbs and knowledge of their use.

It is to be hoped that this guide will not only contribute to the successful treatment of such diseases, but also to a growing return to traditional eating habits and a greater appreciation of the wealth of knowledge that thousands of years of experience with medicinal herbs and foods have left us.

Because to be connected to nature does not only mean to live with it, but also to live from it. To learn from it and to be healed by it. A healing that requires personal initiative as well as the willingness to do without unnatural elements in the diet for the sake of our own organism and its health.

Digestive Herbs
With Recipes according to Hildegard von Bingen

Volume 1 of the book series "World of Herbs"
from the wordsmithery of the Green Archive